BARIATRIC SURGERY RECOVERY DIET

A Comprehensive Guide To Surgery Recovery Diet Plan For Healthy Lifestyle, Weight Maintenance And Vibrant Healing

DR LUCAS KAYCE

DISCLAIMER

This book about illness and nutrition is not meant to replace expert medical advice, diagnosis, or treatment; rather, it is meant purely for informational reasons. This book's content is founded on broad concepts and recommendations for managing diseases and nutrition.

Before adopting any major dietary or lifestyle changes, readers are recommended to speak with a qualified healthcare provider, such as a licensed physician or registered dietitian, especially if they have pre-existing medical concerns. Everybody has different health demands, so what works for one person might not work for another.

The use of the information provided in this book may have unfavorable repercussions or consequences, for which the author and publisher disclaim all liability. No disease is meant to be identified, treated, cured, or prevented by the information provided.

The book may include contain references to medical literature or research findings; however readers are urged to independently confirm this material and contact reliable sources.

It is important to remember that the fields of nutrition and medicine are always changing, and that new findings could have an impact on the advice offered in this book. As a result, readers are urged to keep up with the most recent advancements in healthcare and, when in doubt, seek professional counsel.

By reading this book, readers agree that they are in charge of their own health decisions and release the author and publisher from any liability arising from the use of the material in the book, whether direct or indirect.

TABLE OF CONTENTS

ABOUT THE BOOK

A thorough guide, "Bariatric Surgery Recovery Diet," was written to help people through the crucial post-surgery phase and ensure a long-lasting and successful recovery. This book is crucial because of its careful analysis of the subtleties of bariatric surgery and its provision of a well-organized meal plan that is tailored to the requirements of those undergoing such life-changing operations.

The book explores the basics of bariatric surgery in its first few chapters, stressing the importance of diet after surgery. It explains the rationale behind the recovery diet and serves as an invaluable guide for people who are unfamiliar with the maze of dietary modifications after surgery. The handbook gives readers advice on how to make the most of the material available, enabling them to take control of their rehabilitation process.

The book also discusses the crucial stages of getting ready for bariatric surgery, including consultation, preoperative dietary restrictions, and psychological and mental readiness. By clarifying the various kinds of bariatric operations that are available, it turns into a priceless tool that helps readers choose the procedures that are most suited to their own needs.

The book's primary focus is on the nourishment needed immediately after surgery, taking readers through the phases of clear liquids, full liquids, and pureed foods. It highlights how crucial it is to keep an eye on your food intake and stay hydrated throughout this stage. From then on, the book helps with the smooth transition to solid foods by providing helpful guidance on soft foods, portion control, balanced plate design, and handling key nutrients.

The book adopts a comprehensive stance by offering guidance on maintaining a healthy lifestyle throughout time, even after the initial phase of recovery. It provides advice on how to plan meals, incorporate physical activity, create good eating habits, and identify and deal with emotional eating triggers. Typical problems that people have after surgery are also discussed, along with workable fixes to guarantee a speedy recovery.

The book's deal with how to maintain long-term success, stressing the value of consistent observation, examinations, and networking with like-minded individuals. A useful appendix to the guide offers readers a section with bariatric-friendly recipes for a range of meals, giving them a hands-on way to put the concepts covered in the book into practice.

All things considered, the "Bariatric Surgery Recovery Diet" is an invaluable tool for anyone considering or having bariatric surgery. Its comprehensive methodology, in-depth analyses, and useful suggestions provide it a crucial ally in the pursuit of an effective and long-lasting recuperation following surgery.

AN OVERVIEW OF WEIGHT LOSS SURGERY

In the field of treating obesity and managing weight, bariatric surgery is a quickly developing area that has attracted a lot of interest recently. It is a surgical weight loss method that entails several operations meant to shrink the stomach or change how food is absorbed. Inducing weight loss, resolving obesity-related health problems, and enhancing general quality of life are the main goals of bariatric surgery for patients with morbid obesity.

The wide variety of techniques offered in bariatric surgery, each tailored to unique patient demands and medical conditions, is one of its main features. Gastric bypass, adjustable gastric banding, sleeve gastrectomy, and biliopancreatic diversion with duodenal switch are common operations. These surgical procedures may have a restrictive, malabsorptive, or mixed effect on the body's ability to absorb and utilize nutrients.

The decision to have bariatric surgery is frequently influenced by things like body mass index (BMI), medical disorders linked to obesity, and the ineffectiveness of conventional weight loss techniques.

The importance of a post-surgical diet following bariatric surgery cannot be emphasized. To assist weight loss and prevent nutritional deficiencies, patients' capacity to establish and maintain appropriate food habits is critical to the success of these therapies. To ensure the best possible recovery, encourage long-term weight loss, and manage any issues, post-surgery nutrition is essential. During this stage, patients, medical professionals, and nutritionists must work together to create individualized meal plans that satisfy each person's nutritional needs and adhere to the particular guidelines of the selected bariatric procedure.

THE SIGNIFICANCE OF DIET AFTER SURGERY

Comprehending the significance of nutrition after bariatric surgery entails acknowledging the modified anatomy and physiology that ensue from the procedure.

It is important to carefully evaluate nutrient intake because patients frequently suffer changes in dietary tolerance, appetite, and nutrient absorption.

Not only is healthy eating important for maintaining a healthy weight, but it also helps avoid vitamin and mineral shortages. Sufficient consumption of protein is especially important for maintaining muscle mass and accelerating the body's healing process following surgery.

Furthermore, by assisting patients in sticking to their weight loss objectives and enhancing their general well-being, post-surgery nutrition adds to the long-term success of bariatric therapies. Making the switch to a healthier lifestyle includes not just eating a different diet but also getting regular exercise and dealing with food-related behaviors.

Patients are urged to adopt whole foods, portion control, and mindful eating techniques as part of a sustainable and well-rounded nutritional approach.

Bariatric surgery is a life-changing experience for anyone looking for long-term, practical answers to their obesity. The variety of surgical techniques that are accessible emphasizes the value of individualized treatment, with post-surgery nutrition standing out as essential to recovery. A dedication to dietary modifications, strict attention to nutritional requirements, and continuous support from medical professionals is necessary for navigating the post-operative phase. The development of comprehensive post-surgical dietary regimens is crucial to improving general health and optimizing results for patients undergoing bariatric surgery, as the area of this transformative operation continues to progress.

CHAPTER ONE

GETTING READY FOR YOUR GASTRIC PROCEDURE

CONSULTATION AND ASSESSMENT

Individuals usually go through a thorough consultation and evaluation process before having bariatric surgery. This entails scheduling consultations with medical specialists like psychologists, dietitians, and surgeons to evaluate the patient's general health and establish if they qualify for the treatment. During the appointment, all worries or inquiries from the patient can be addressed and a full discussion of the possible advantages and dangers of bariatric surgery can take place. In this phase, the surgical technique is customized for each patient based on their medical history, current health, and lifestyle factors.

GUIDELINES FOR PREOPERATIVE DIET

Following recommended diet requirements before to bariatric surgery is an essential part of the preparation process. By assisting patients in reducing their body weight and liver size, these guidelines aim to improve the safety and effectiveness of surgical treatment.

A high-protein, low-carb diet is usually part of the preoperative diet to encourage weight loss and reduce the possibility of surgical complications. Adhering to these dietary guidelines helps to promote long-term weight management, aid in postoperative recovery, and make surgery go more smoothly.

PSYCHOLOGICAL AND EMOTIONAL READINESS

There is more to being physically ready for bariatric surgery than just being mentally and emotionally prepared. Many people who are considering bariatric surgery have experienced difficulties connected to their weight and emotional eating.

To assist patients in addressing underlying emotional difficulties and developing coping mechanisms, psychosocial assessments and counseling sessions are frequently included in the initial phase of care. To improve the patient's long-term outcomes and general well-being, this mental and emotional preparation attempts to increase the patient's resilience, motivation, and commitment to the lifestyle adjustments that come with bariatric surgery.

MODIFICATIONS IN LIFESTYLE

Significant lifestyle changes are brought about by bariatric surgery, and it is crucial to plan for these adjustments to have a positive outcome.

To aid in their weight loss efforts, patients are urged to take up healthy routines including mindful eating and frequent exercise. Modifying eating habits, controlling portions, and cultivating a healthy relationship with food are other aspects of changing one's lifestyle. Postoperative assistance helps patients adjust to these lifestyle adjustments successfully. Examples of this assistance include involvement in support groups and nutritional advice.

Maintaining weight loss and improving general health following bariatric surgery need a sustained commitment to these lifestyle changes and an acceptance of a holistic approach to health and well-being.

CHAPTER TWO

RECOGNIZING THE TYPES OF BARIATRIC SURGERY

GASTRIC BYPASS

One kind of bariatric surgery called a gastric bypass entails rerouting the digestive system and producing a tiny stomach pouch. The small intestine is connected to both the smaller upper and larger lower sections of the stomach when the surgeon separates them. This alteration affects how much food the stomach can store and how the small intestine absorbs nutrients. Patients suffer from decreased food intake and malabsorption as a result, which causes them to lose a lot of weight. Gastric bypass surgery is one of the most popular bariatric treatments because of its reputation for facilitating significant and long-lasting weight loss.

GASTRECTOMY WITH SLEEVE

A major piece of the stomach is removed during a sleeve gastrectomy, sometimes referred to as gastric sleeve surgery, leaving behind a device that resembles a banana or sleeve. This technique makes the stomach smaller, which limits the quantity of food it can hold and makes smaller meals feel fuller. In addition, the portion of the stomach that produces the hunger hormone ghrelin is removed after surgery, which also reduces appetite. Because it can lead to significant weight loss and has a lower risk of problems than some other procedures, sleeve gastrectomy is a popular procedure.

ADJUSTABLE GASTRIC BANDING

An inflated silicone band is wrapped around the top portion of the stomach during adjustable gastric banding, often known as lap-band surgery. By forming a little pouch, this band limits how much food the stomach can hold and slows down the digesting process. Through a port positioned just below the skin, saline solution can be injected into or removed from the band to modify it. This setting gives you individual control over the band's tightness and the speed at which you lose weight. Adjustable gastric banding is thought to be less intrusive than other bariatric surgeries, however, the amount of weight lost may not be as great.

DIVERSION OF THE BILIOPANCREAS USING DUODENAL SWITCH

The intricate bariatric procedure known as biliopancreatic diversion with duodenal switch (BPD/DS) consists of two parts. To start, the stomach is made smaller using a sleeve gastrectomy. Then, a large section of the small intestine is skipped, which modifies the way nutrients are absorbed.

This dual mechanism causes significant weight loss by having malabsorptive and restrictive effects. For people with obesity-related health problems and a higher body mass index (BMI), BPD/DS is usually advised. On the other hand, there is a greater chance of nutritional inadequacies, necessitating ongoing monitoring and supplementation.

SELECTING THE BEST PROCESS FOR YOU

It is important to carefully evaluate individual aspects including BMI, general health, lifestyle, and personal preferences before choosing the best bariatric operation. For anyone looking for a more drastic method of weight loss and those with a higher BMI, gastric bypass is frequently advised. Because of its effectiveness and decreased risk profile, sleeve gastrectomy is appropriate for a large number of people. If you would rather have a less intrusive option where you can modify the band, you might want to think about adjustable gastric banding. Usually, BPD/DS is saved for particular situations where a more involved process is required. The finest bariatric surgery can be chosen for each patient after speaking with a healthcare provider and going through a thorough evaluation. This will assist in ensuring the greatest results for long-term weight loss and general health.

CHAPTER THREE

QUICK POST-OPERATIVE NUTRITION

PHASE OF CLEAR LIQUIDS

The first few days following surgery are critical for the body's healing and recuperation. A gradual return to a regular diet is ensured by introducing several phases, with nutrition playing a crucial part during this time.

Clear Liquids Phase is the initial stage of post-surgery nutrition. Patients are only allowed to drink clear liquids at this point, including broth, water, and clear juices. This stage keeps the body from becoming dehydrated and gives it the vital fluids it needs without overtaxing the digestive system. Because they are readily absorbed, clear beverages help to maintain fluid balance and prevent problems.

COMPLETE PHASE OF LIQUIDS

The Full Liquids Phase comes after the Clear Liquids Phase. More substantial liquids, including milk, soups, and other liquid-based foods, are introduced at this period. Full liquids give the body the extra calories and nutrients it needs to meet its energy requirements while it heals. For people who may still find it difficult to eat solid foods but require more nutrition than clear liquids can provide, this stage is crucial.

MAKING THE SWITCH TO PUREED FOODS

Transitioning to Pureed Foods is the next stage when patients become better. Pureed foods are simple to digest and aid in a person's return to a somewhat regular diet. Foods in this phase are usually pureed to a smooth consistency to facilitate simpler digestion and ingestion. Foods that have been pureed offer more nutrients with minimal impact on the digestive tract.

TRACKING NUTRITION CONSUMPTION

One of the most important aspects of post-surgery nutrition is tracking nutrient consumption. Sufficient amounts of protein, vitamins, and minerals are necessary for the body to recover itself. For example, protein is essential for the immune system and tissue healing. To make sure they satisfy their unique dietary demands during the recovery phase, patients should collaborate closely with healthcare providers or dietitians. Continual evaluations and dietary modifications can be required depending on how each person responds to the various stages.

MAINTAINING HYDRATION

It's critical to maintain fluid intake for the duration of the recovery period following surgery. Maintaining adequate hydration promotes several physiological processes, helps avoid problems, and speeds up the healing process. When solid foods are prohibited during the first clear liquids phase, it is extremely important to consume enough fluids. Urine color and output monitoring is a straightforward but reliable method of determining one's level of hydration.

Understanding the various stages of a post-surgery diet is critical to a full recovery. Without overtaxing the digestive system, the steady transition from clear liquids to full liquids and finally to pureed foods restores its functionality. Keeping an eye on your nutritional intake and drinking plenty of water are essential parts of this process, which guarantees the body gets the support it needs for the best possible healing and recuperation following surgery.

CHAPTER FOUR

TRANSITIONING GRADUALLY TO SOLID FOODS

OVERVIEW OF SOFT FOODS

One of the most important life milestones is moving from a liquid to a solid diet, especially in the early stages of infancy. The introduction of soft foods is the first step toward a diet that is more varied and complex. The transition from solely consuming breast milk or formula to a broader range of nutrients necessary for growth and development is facilitated by soft meals. To guarantee a seamless and easy transition for the person, much attention must be paid to the texture, consistency, and nutritional value of meals.

ASSEMBLING AN EQUILIBRIUM PLATE

When babies and young kids start eating solid foods, it's critical to concentrate on creating a plate that is balanced and contains a range of nutrients. A well-balanced dish has an assortment of proteins, carbs, fats, vitamins, and minerals. Including a wide variety of soft meals contributes to a balanced nutritional profile that supports the growth of different body functions. Planning and preparing meals that support a child's general health and well-being from an early age is a critical responsibility of parents and other caregivers.

STRATEGIES FOR PORTION CONTROL

A crucial component of the gradual switch to solid foods is portion control. To avoid overindulging and maintain a balanced calorie intake, it is crucial to control portion sizes as children start to experiment with different textures and flavors.

Offering serving sizes that are appropriate for the child's age, size, and developmental stage is one of the portion control tactics. This promotes the development of mindful eating practices that will benefit the person for the rest of their life and aid in the prevention of any digestive problems.

THE VALUE OF CONSUMING PROTEIN

Since protein is essential for growth and development, it plays a key role in the transition to solid foods. Soft foods high in protein support the growth of muscles, the healing of damaged tissue, and the body's general operation. Including protein sources in the diet, such as dairy, lentils, and soft meats, guarantees that the youngster eats enough of the important amino acids. Parents need to introduce a range of soft foods that are high in protein to their children to assist their physical development and meet their nutritional needs.

TAKING CARE OF MINERALS AND VITAMINS

Soft meals can also be an excellent way to get important minerals and vitamins that are needed for several bodily functions. Including a variety of fruits, vegetables, and fortified cereals helps to supply a range of vitamins and minerals that are essential for immune system function, bone health, and general well-being. When their child is gradually moving from soft to solid foods, parents should think about the nutritional value of soft foods and make educated decisions to guarantee that the child gets a balanced intake of vitamins and minerals.

The introduction of soft foods represents a critical turning point in the formation of a person's eating habits. A balanced plate, portion control techniques, a focus on protein consumption, and vitamin and mineral management are all crucial elements of this shift. Caregivers can help lay a wholesome and nourishing foundation for lifelong healthy eating habits by carefully managing these factors.

CHAPTER FIVE

DEVELOPING A SUSTAINABLE DIET PLAN

DEVELOPING HEALTHFUL EATING PRACTICES

Developing good eating habits is the first step in creating a sustainable diet plan. It entails making deliberate decisions to eat a wholesome, well-balanced diet that satisfies the body's needs for optimum operation. Focusing on complete, unprocessed foods like fruits, vegetables, whole grains, lean meats, and healthy fats is important. These foods support general health and supply vital nutrients.

Portion control is another essential component. Gaining knowledge about portion sizes promotes weight management by preventing overeating. Including a range of foods in meals guarantees a wide range of nutrients, promoting a more nutritious and well-balanced diet. Furthermore, mindful eating encourages a better relationship with food and reduces needless calorie consumption by paying attention to signals of hunger and fullness.

TIPS FOR MEAL PLANNING AND PREPARATION

A sustainable eating plan must include efficient meal planning and preparation. Meal preparation in advance enables people to choose better options, waste less food, and save time. It entails planning a weekly menu, taking dietary requirements into account, and including a variety of foods. Batch cooking is a useful tactic because it allows you to prepare several meals at once, which saves you time every week.

When it comes to grocery shopping, favoring fresh, seasonal produce and eliminating processed foods boosts the nutritional content of meals. Reading food labels can aid in making informed choices, considering variables such as added sugars and preservatives. Additionally, involving the whole family in meal preparation can make the process more fun and encourage a sense of shared responsibility for keeping a good eating regimen.

INCORPORATING PHYSICAL ACTIVITY

A sustainable eating plan goes hand in hand with frequent physical activity. Engaging in exercise not only contributes to weight management but also supports general health and well-being. Combining a balanced diet with physical activity helps maintain a healthy body weight, promotes cardiovascular health, and boosts metabolism.

Incorporating numerous sorts of workouts, including aerobic activities, strength training, and flexibility exercises, ensures a holistic approach to fitness. Finding activities that are enjoyable increases the likelihood of long-term adherence. Whether it's walking, cycling, swimming, or participating in group classes, the key is to establish a routine that aligns with individual preferences and fits into daily life.

RECOGNIZING EMOTIONAL EATING TRIGGERS:

Emotional eating is a common challenge that can undermine a sustainable eating plan. It involves using food as a coping mechanism for emotional stress, boredom, or other feelings. Recognizing emotional eating triggers is essential for developing a healthier relationship with food. Identifying situations, emotions, or stressors that lead to emotional eating allows individuals to implement alternative coping strategies.

Mindfulness practices, such as meditation and deep breathing, can help manage stress and reduce the likelihood of turning to food for comfort. Seeking support from friends, family, or a mental health professional can also be beneficial in addressing the underlying emotional issues that contribute to emotional eating. Developing a mindful approach to eating, where individuals are present and attentive during meals, further aids in breaking the cycle of emotional eating and promotes a sustainable, balanced lifestyle.

CHAPTER SIX

COMMON CHALLENGES AND SOLUTIONS

DEALING WITH FOOD INTOLERANCES

Navigating food intolerances can be a challenging aspect of maintaining a healthy lifestyle. Individuals with food intolerances may experience adverse reactions to certain foods, leading to discomfort and potential health issues. Identifying and managing these intolerances requires a personalized approach. Elimination diets, where specific foods are removed from the diet and gradually reintroduced, can help pinpoint triggers.

Working with a registered dietitian can provide valuable guidance, as they can create a tailored nutrition plan that ensures essential nutrients are not compromised while avoiding problematic foods. Additionally, food labels should be scrutinized, and alternative ingredients sought to maintain a balanced and varied diet, promoting overall well-being.

ADDRESSING NUTRIENT DEFICIENCIES

Nutrient deficiencies can significantly impact health and well-being, posing challenges for individuals striving to maintain optimal nutritional status. Identifying and addressing these deficiencies is crucial to prevent potential health complications. Regular monitoring through blood tests can aid in the early detection of deficiencies. Supplementation, under the guidance of healthcare professionals, may be necessary to bridge nutritional gaps. A balanced diet rich in diverse fruits, vegetables, lean proteins, and whole grains is foundational to preventing deficiencies. Collaborating with a registered dietitian can help individuals tailor their diets to meet specific nutritional needs, ensuring a comprehensive and sustainable approach to addressing deficiencies.

COPING WITH PLATEAUS

Experiencing plateaus in health and fitness journeys is a common challenge that can be demotivating. Plateaus occur when progress stalls, whether in weight loss, fitness gains, or other health-related goals. It's essential to recognize that plateaus are a natural part of the process, and adapting strategies is key to overcoming them. Incorporating variety into workouts, adjusting the intensity and duration of exercises, and reassessing dietary habits can help break through plateaus. Setting realistic and achievable goals, celebrating small victories, and staying consistent with healthy habits contribute to sustained progress. Seeking support from peers, fitness communities, or professionals can provide valuable insights and motivation during challenging plateaus.

SEEKING SUPPORT FROM HEALTHCARE PROFESSIONALS

Engaging with healthcare professionals is a fundamental aspect of achieving and maintaining optimal health. Whether addressing specific health concerns, managing chronic conditions, or seeking guidance on lifestyle changes, healthcare professionals play a crucial role.

Establishing open communication with primary care physicians, specialists, and registered dietitians is essential for receiving personalized advice and treatment plans. Regular health check-ups, screenings, and consultations can aid in early detection and prevention of potential issues. Building a collaborative relationship with healthcare providers fosters a supportive environment for individuals to make informed decisions about their health and well-being. Seeking professional guidance ensures that interventions are evidence-based and tailored to individual needs, promoting a holistic approach to health and longevity.

CHAPTER SEVEN

MAINTAINING LONG-TERM SUCCESS

REGULAR MONITORING AND CHECK-UPS

Regular monitoring and check-ups are crucial components in maintaining long-term success, particularly in endeavors such as weight management or post-bariatric surgery care. Continuous oversight allows individuals to track their progress, identify potential challenges, and make necessary adjustments to their lifestyle. Regular check-ups with healthcare professionals, nutritionists, or support groups provide an opportunity to assess physical health, nutritional intake, and emotional well-being. This proactive approach helps in the early detection of issues, ensuring timely interventions and sustained success.

ADJUSTING TO LIFE AFTER BARIATRIC SURGERY

Adjusting to life after bariatric surgery is a multifaceted process that extends beyond the operating room. It involves adapting to new dietary habits, addressing emotional changes, and embracing a transformed lifestyle. Patients often encounter challenges as they navigate through these adjustments, such as understanding portion control, adopting mindful eating habits, and incorporating regular physical activity. Seeking guidance from healthcare professionals, attending post-surgery support groups, and working closely with dieticians can significantly aid individuals in overcoming these challenges and promoting long-term success.

BUILDING A SUPPORTIVE NETWORK

Building a supportive network is instrumental in maintaining long-term success, especially in endeavors that require lifestyle changes. Whether it is weight management or recovery after bariatric surgery, having a strong support system can provide emotional encouragement, practical assistance, and a sense of community. Family, friends, and support groups play vital roles in offering understanding, motivation, and accountability. Sharing experiences, discussing challenges, and receiving encouragement from others who have undergone similar journeys fosters a sense of belonging, making the path to long-term success more sustainable.

CELEBRATING MILESTONES

Celebrating milestones is an integral aspect of sustaining motivation and reinforcing positive behavior. Whether it's losing a certain amount of weight, reaching a fitness goal, or adhering to dietary recommendations, acknowledging and celebrating achievements helps individuals stay motivated and committed to their long-term objectives.

Recognizing milestones can be a powerful reinforcement mechanism, boosting self-esteem and fostering a positive mindset. This positive reinforcement contributes to the overall success by creating a sense of accomplishment and further motivating individuals to continue their journey towards sustained well-being.

Maintaining long-term success in areas such as weight management or post-bariatric surgery care involves a holistic approach. Regular monitoring and check-ups provide a foundation for ongoing assessment and necessary adjustments. Adapting to life after surgery requires a comprehensive understanding of lifestyle changes, emotional adjustments, and support systems. Building a supportive network is essential for emotional encouragement and practical assistance. Celebrating milestones serves as a positive reinforcement mechanism, enhancing motivation and fostering a sustained commitment to long-term success. By incorporating these concepts into one's journey, individuals can create a robust framework for achieving and maintaining their health and wellness goals over the long term.

CHAPTER EIGHT

RECIPES FOR BARIATRIC-FRIENDLY MEALS

BREAKFAST IDEAS

For individuals undergoing bariatric surgery or those focusing on weight management, breakfast is a crucial meal to kick start the day with nutrient-dense options that provide sustained energy. Opting for protein-rich breakfasts can help keep you satiated and maintain muscle mass. Consider incorporating eggs, Greek yogurt, or protein smoothies made with low-fat milk or plant-based alternatives. These options not only provide essential proteins but also offer a variety of textures and flavors to keep your mornings interesting.

Another excellent choice for a bariatric-friendly breakfast is oatmeal. Rich in fiber, it promotes a feeling of fullness and supports digestive health. Customize your oatmeal with fruits, nuts, and a drizzle of honey for added taste without compromising on nutritional value. Additionally, whole-grain options like quinoa or whole wheat toast can be integrated, ensuring a balance of carbohydrates to fuel your day.

LUNCH AND DINNER RECIPES

When crafting bariatric-friendly lunch and dinner recipes, focus on lean proteins, vegetables, and whole grains. Grilled chicken or fish, paired with colorful vegetables like broccoli, spinach, and bell peppers, make for satisfying and nutritious meals. Consider incorporating quinoa, brown rice, or sweet potatoes to add complex carbohydrates, which release energy gradually.

Experiment with flavorful herbs and spices to enhance taste without relying on excessive fats or sugars. Utilizing techniques like roasting, grilling, or steaming helps retain the natural goodness of ingredients without adding unnecessary calories. Portion control is crucial, and dividing meals into smaller, more frequent servings throughout the day can assist in better digestion and absorption of nutrients.

For a lighter alternative, salads with a variety of veggies, lean proteins, and a vinaigrette dressing provide a refreshing option. Explore different protein sources like tofu, beans, or legumes for plant-based alternatives that are both satisfying and nutrient-packed.

SNACKS AND DESSERTS

Smart snacking is essential for individuals managing weight or undergoing bariatric surgery. Opt for snacks that combine protein with healthy fats or fiber to keep you feeling full between meals. Nuts, seeds, and Greek yogurt with a drizzle of honey are excellent choices. Additionally, consider fresh fruit or vegetables with hummus for a satisfying and nutritious snack.

When it comes to desserts, moderation is key. Explore recipes that use alternatives to refined sugars, such as natural sweeteners like stevia or monk fruit. Fruit-based desserts, like baked apples or berry compotes, can satisfy a sweet tooth while providing essential vitamins and antioxidants.

Mindfully incorporating small indulgences ensures that you can enjoy dessert without compromising your health goals.

SAMPLE MEAL PLANS

Creating balanced and bariatric-friendly meal plans involves a thoughtful combination of macronutrients and micronutrients. A typical day might start with a protein-rich breakfast, such as scrambled eggs with spinach and a side of Greek yogurt.

For lunch, a grilled chicken salad with a variety of colorful vegetables and a light vinaigrette dressing can provide essential nutrients without excess calories.

Afternoon snacks may include a handful of nuts or a protein smoothie to maintain energy levels. Dinner could consist of baked fish with quinoa and roasted vegetables. For dessert, a small serving of a fruit-based option like a mixed berry parfait or a baked apple can offer a satisfying end to the day.

It's crucial to stay hydrated throughout the day, so incorporate water and herbal teas into your routine. Adjust portion sizes based on individual needs and consult with a healthcare professional or nutritionist to personalize meal plans according to specific dietary requirements and health goals.

www.ingramcontent.com/pod-product-compliance
Lightning Source LLC
Chambersburg PA
CBHW060815260726
48660CB00002B/964